Cataract Surgery Handbook

**A Guide to Successful Cataract Surgery
in the Daytona Beach Area**

**2nd edition
2021**

Written and Illustrated by
the Tomoka Eye Doctors

www.TomokaEye.com

CONTENTS

～ Welcome ～

Tomoka "Eye-Toons"

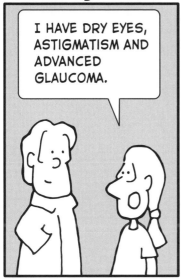

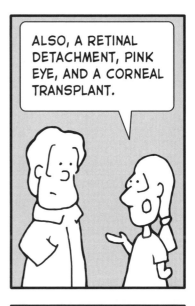

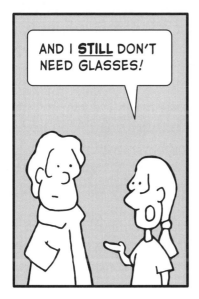

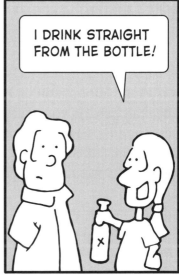

Do you have a cataract?

If you are reading this little book, you must have visited us and we must have discussed cataracts and cataract surgery.

Cataract surgery is the most common adult surgical procedure performed in the United States, and one of the most successful. This procedure has improved the vision and quality of life for millions of Americans. However, the prospect of eye surgery is scary for most people and you probably have questions.

Questions like:
>What is a cataract again?
>Do I really need surgery?
>What will I experience during my surgery?
>Am I going to need glasses afterward?

We attempt to answer these questions during your office visit, but many questions may occur to you AFTER you leave. To eliminate confusion, and hopefully alleviate some of your anxiety, we've created this little book of answers. Here you will find an exhaustive list of questions that people ask us ... questions before, during, and after their surgery.

This is a lot of information and we don't want you to feel like you HAVE to read this. If you have concerns that aren't addressed within these pages, or don't feel like searching, please call our office. If our surgical coordinators and technicians can't answer your inquiry, we'll be happy to call you and go over things personally.

This book is a work in progress. We are continually expanding and adding content, so please pardon the grammar and typographical errors you may find.

We hope you find this information useful. Your eyes are important, and we want to make sure you are completely informed before considering an operation! Thanks so much!

The Tomoka Eye Doctors

Disclaimers

1

If you see another doctor (outside of our practice), you may find information in this book that conflicts with what you've been told about cataracts. When in doubt, listen to the doctor who has actually seen your eyes in person. This book reflects our own personal beliefs, surgical experiences, and is specific to the greater Daytona Beach area.

2

To keep this book interesting, we've added many cartoons and comic strips. These silly jokes are not meant to downplay eye disease or disrespect our patients. Rather, this lighthearted approach is meant to keep this book palatable and easy to read. We mean no offense, and hope you approach these cartoons with the same good-natured outlook that we had when we illustrated them.

3

This book is not meant to 'replace' the normal consent process of surgery. We will talk to you at great length about cataracts during your consultation visit in our office - and you should ask us questions! Consider this book supplemental education.

4

Surgical technology is advancing rapidly and some of the content within these pages may become dated with time. For example, "laser cataract surgery" was unproven a few years ago and barely discussed in the last version of this book. Today, laser surgery has a proven track record and is commonplace. Future advances in implant design and post-operative drug delivery may make some of the following chapters obsolete in a few years.

Chapter 1

⤷ Introduction ↺

Tomoka "Eye-Toons"

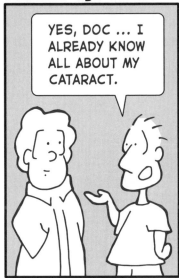

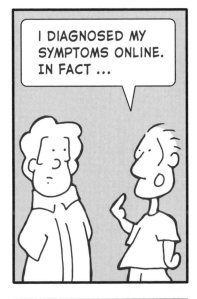

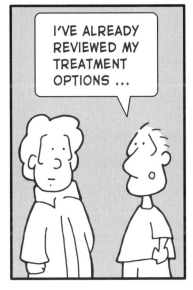

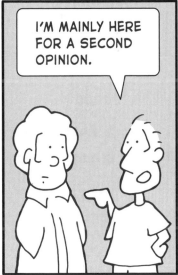

Introduction to Cataracts

Do you need surgery?

What exactly is a cataract?

When the lens inside your eye becomes cloudy, you have a cataract. This cloudiness develops gradually with age and can create glare or blurry vision. A cataract makes it harder for you to distinguish distant objects or read small print.

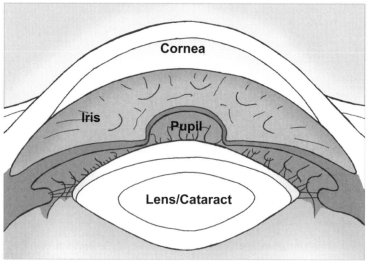

A cataract is a cloudy lens inside your eye.

There is a lens inside my eye?

Yes. Inside the eye sits a "magnifying glass" called the lens. This lens is suspended behind our iris (the colored part of the eye). When light enters the eye, it passes through the dark pupil and through this lens before reaching the retina at the back of the eye.

If your lens becomes cloudy (a cataract), light has difficulty reaching the retina and your vision is affected.

How does my "lens" become cloudy and turn into a cataract?

The clear lens inside your eye is living tissue, and over your lifetime, cloudy proteins form within this clear tissue. These proteins obstruct light and create a "haziness" to the clear lens. When the haziness is bad enough to be detected, we start calling this a "cataract."

Most cataracts form as part of the normal aging process. The cloudy proteins accumulate over time as a result of the natural metabolism occurring inside the eye. In fact, everyone over the age of 40 has some mild cataract formation, though it usually takes several decades for the cataract to become visually significant.

But I'm not that old! Can cataracts form in younger people?

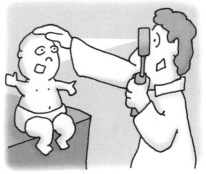

While we normally think of cataracts as an eye problem in the older population, some people develop them much earlier. This early maturation can sometimes have a genetic inheritance pattern. Metabolism changes in the body, such as diabetes or steroid use, can cause early cataracts. Cataracts can develop years after a forgotten eye injury as well. Even infants can be born with congenital cataracts and require surgery to avoid permanent vision loss.

Is there anything I can do to avoid cataracts or make mine go away?

Not really. For most people, cataract formation is a normal aging process inside the eye. There is not much you can do to slow this process down, other than wearing sunglasses to reduce UV exposure. There has been research on oral medications and eye drops that might slow cataract formation, but the results have been unconvincing and the "successes" questionable. The only way to get rid of a cataract is surgical removal.

Can my medication cause my cataracts?

The main medications associated with early cataract formation are steroids. If you take a topical, oral, or inhaled steroid (for asthma, for instance) this can lead to clouding of the lens.

What are the symptoms of my cataract?

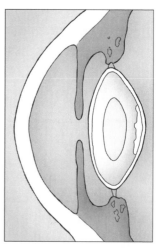

The first symptom that most people describe to us is one of glare . . . especially at night. For example, you might find nighttime driving challenging because of halos you see around the headlights of oncoming traffic.

Other people don't have this glare problem because they "just don't drive that much at night, anyway!" Instead, their cataract causes more problems with visual "crispness" and difficulty seeing fine detail. For example, you might have a hard time reading small print or seeing distant road signs, despite your eyeglasses being up-to-date.

Why do my eyeglass prescriptions keep changing?

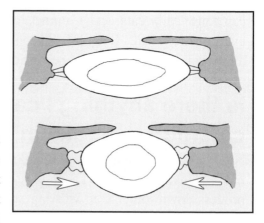

Remember, a cataract/lens is like a magnifying glass inside your eye. As the cataract worsens, the strength of that magnifying glass changes and this affects your eye's overall focus power. This can lead to rapid changes in your eyeglass prescription.

How can I tell if my cataract is getting worse?

For most people, a worsening cataract becomes obvious with deteriorating vision. If you are having more difficulties with night vision, or with reading small words on your television, this could be from a worsening cataract.

Many cataracts form slowly and your visual blur might not be obvious. If your vision loss is gradual, you may not notice how poor your vision has gotten until it is far gone. When we check your vision in the office, we can track how your vision changes over time and give you a better sense of how you're doing compared to past visits.

Can you judge my cataract by looking at my eyes in the office?

We can see your cataract by examining your eyes under a microscope. A cataract looks cloudy with a yellow tint that glows brightly when illuminated by a beam of light.

While a cataract is easy to detect with a microscope, the SEVERITY of your cataract is harder to judge. We can't always determine whether a cataract "needs to come out" by our microscopic examination alone. We are always amazed by "wimpy looking" cataracts that seem to cause major vision problems. And yet, some patients have cataracts that look "horrendous" under the microscope but still have good vision.

When it comes down to it, it really isn't just what the DOCTOR sees when looking at your eyes that matters. What matters is how well

YOU see in your daily activities. Your opinion is important in helping make this decision.

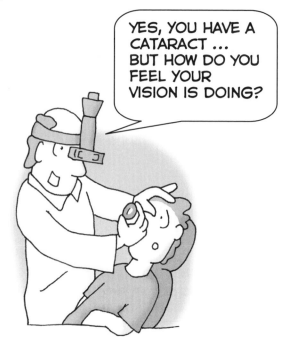

YES, YOU HAVE A CATARACT ...
BUT HOW DO YOU FEEL YOUR VISION IS DOING?

How can you tell if a cataract is causing glare?

We can estimate glare problems by checking your vision in a dark room using an eyechart. We then RECHECK your vision using glare-inducing lights. If your vision worsens under these conditions, then we know glare must be causing problems out in the "wild" as well.

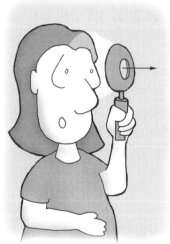

Checking for glare problems using the "Brightness Acuity Tester"

How do I know if I need cataract surgery?

This really is the big question, right? Should your cataract come out? Will surgery be worth it? Do you really need to subject yourself to an operation? Just because we CAN remove a cataract, doesn't necessarily mean we MUST remove it immediately.

The only downside to this hands-off philosophy is that the longer we wait for a cataract to develop, the "harder" the cataract becomes. The cataract lens can become physically dense and hard like a rock! A dense, hard cataract may increase some risk factors during and after surgery.

The key for YOU is to deal with your cataract once it "ripens," but before it gets "too dense." For most people, than means waiting until your vision starts to worsen such that your lifestyle becomes affected (you don't feel safe driving at night, for example). Just like everything else in life, it's about balancing the benefits with the risks . . . and deciding when the time is "right" for surgery is not always obvious.

Are there times when you recommend cataract surgery despite your patient having no major vision complaints?

On rare occasions, we'll recommend cataract surgery even if you don't have any significant vision problems. This is usually because:

1. Your cataract is looking extremely dense and we're worried about complications with delayed surgery.

2. Your pupils don't dilate well and your cataract is advancing quickly.

3. Your cataract is causing other problems, such as glaucoma.

4. You need your cataract removed before you can have another surgery (such as retina surgery).

These situations don't arise very often, and we don't push for surgery unless we really believe it necessary. Remember, cataract surgery is an elective surgery ... and when it comes to elective surgeries, the goal is to minimize risk.

I trust you ... you're the doctor. You just tell me when I should have my cataract surgery!

We're sure you have many complex problems in your life and other issues take precedence over your vision. It would be nice to let your doctor tell you when "the time is right" for cataract surgery. Unfortunately, we just can't make this decision for you.

Once upon a time, your doctor told you what to do, and you followed instructions. However, healthcare has changed. The biggest advocate for your own health is now YOU, and you need to have a reasonable understanding of your treatment options if you want to have reasonable outcomes.

Our job is to educate and give you the tools to help you make an intelligent decision about potential cataract surgery. Then, our responsibility is to do a good job and support you through this experience.

We promise to do our best to gauge the severity of your cataract and educate you about what kind of visual improvements to expect. We'll even tell you whether "we feel" the benefits of surgery outweigh the risks in your particular case.

But remember . . . despite all safety precautions and the best surgical intentions, unexpected things can happen.

Are you any good at this?

We think we're pretty good at cataract surgery . . . like most ophthalmologists, cataract surgery is our primary surgery and each of our doctors currently performs 10-20 cataract surgeries in a day. Tomoka Eye has been performing cataract surgery in the Daytona Beach area for more than 40 years. We all have good eyes, steady hands, and are risk-averse. However, we make no claims at being superhuman.

Cataract surgery is the "most common" operation for our ophthalmologists. We do this surgery thousands and thousands of times. Just like any other task . . . be it cooking, golf, or juggling chainsaws . . . you can't help but get good and develop proficiency when you do something this often.

Are you experienced enough to be doing cataract surgery on me?

Picking your surgeon can be a nerve-wracking experience, especially when your eye doctor looks younger than your children.

We like to think of ophthalmologists falling along an "experience spectrum." On one end, you have younger doctors who trained using the most modern equipment and who have (at least theoretically) good hands, eyes and reflexes for this kind of delicate procedure. On the other end of the spectrum, you have older eye doctors who trained via older methods, but kept themselves up-to-date with modern techniques and have the wisdom of experience.

Quite frankly, we feel that ALL the eye doctors in the Daytona Beach area are very good and all of them will do a great job for you.

The biggest key for YOU is to find an eye doctor that you are comfortable with, who you feel confident in, and who you feel will do right by you in the unlikely event that your surgical path is a little rocky.

How is cataract surgery performed?

Cataract surgery is a procedure that involves removing the cloudy cataract from your eye and replacing it with a clear lens implant. This procedure takes only 15 minutes. You are awake throughout the procedure, but we do place an IV in your arm so that we can give you pain relaxing medicines (if you need any). You can't see the instruments during the surgery, just a bright light from the microscope.

To get your cataract out, we need to physically remove it. The OLD way of performing cataract surgery involved making a very LARGE incision and removing the cataract in one big giant piece. We would then sew numerous stitches in your eye and the visual recovery would take months and involve tedious suture removal. Today, we perform this surgery through a TINY microincision that is so small it seals on its own with little eye irritation and usually no stitches at all!

Once we've created the microincision into the eye, we remove the cataract tissue by breaking it up into small pieces and vacuuming these pieces out with a delicate ultrasonic device.

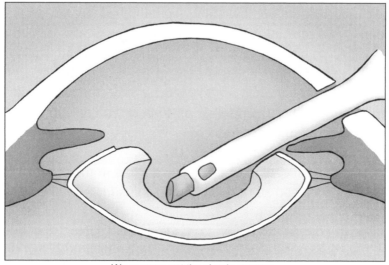

We vacuum out the cloudy cataract.

We then inject a new "implant" back into the eye. This implanted lens folds, allowing us to inject it through the microincision. Once inside the eye, the implant unfolds like a blossoming flower and replaces your cataract with a nice clear lens.

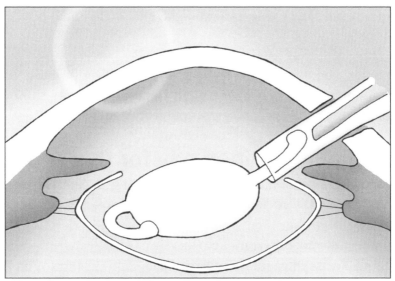

A new implant lens is placed back inside the eye.

After your implant is in secure position, we sit you up. We then give you coffee/tea and a muffin to fill your empty stomach while we review your post-operative instructions. We then send you home the same morning. You'll use eye drops at home and wear a clear shield taped over your eye at bedtime and while napping.

Do you use needles or stitches in my eye?

Normally, no. We use an IV in your arm to give you pain medications and an eye drop anesthesia to numb the eye, so that needles aren't needed near your eye!

The microincision made is so small (2.7 millimeters) that you don't feel it, and it seals up on its own after surgery without the need for stitches.

What kind of vision should I expect after cataract surgery?

The purpose of cataract surgery is to make your vision clearer, crisper, and to reduce glare. This will make it easier to perform fine tasks like threading a needle, driving a car at night, and seeing small print on the television screen.

Sometimes, you don't need glasses at all (at least for distance vision), but that's more of a secondary benefit - and most people still benefit from wearing a mild eyeglass prescription after surgery.

Does my insurance pay for this?

Just about every private insurance, including Medicare, pays for cataract surgery since this is a medical diagnosis. Your insurance covers:

- Cataract Surgeon's Fee (that's us!)
- Facility Fee (our surgery center)
- Standard Implant
- Follow-up Care

Your insurance does not pay for deductibles, co-pays, laser surgery, or for the "premium" implants. Our surgery coordinator will answer your questions about out-of-pocket expenses and specifics.

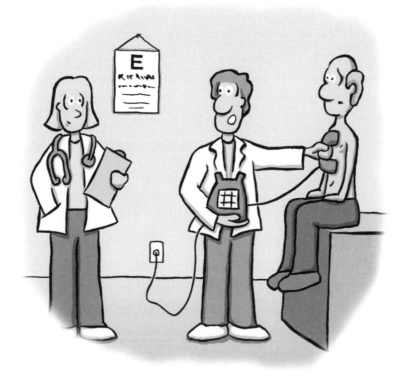

"His cardiologist is on vacation,
so we're leaving a message."

Chapter 2
❧ Implants & Measurements ❧

Tomoka "Eye-Toons"

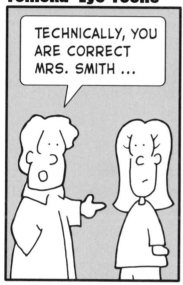

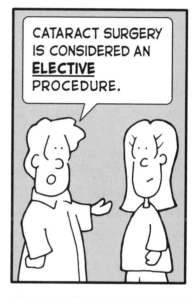

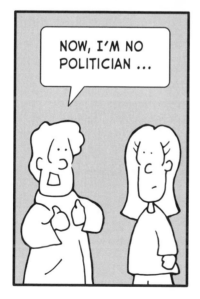

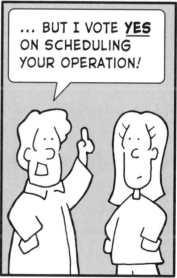

Implants & Measurements

Whether you'll need glasses after surgery

During cataract surgery, we place an implant inside your eye. This implant is crystal clear and gives you crisp vision. These implants also come in different prescriptions and can drastically reduce your dependence on glasses after surgery. But, before we get into details, let's start with the basics.

What exactly is an implant?

The "implant" is the plastic lens that we place inside your eye. When we remove your cataract, a new lens has to go back inside to replace it. Without a new lens, you wouldn't be able to see. Before lens implants were invented, people had to use coke-bottle glasses after cataract surgery to get around.

The modern implants we use are made of a flexible acrylic plastic. These plastic lenses are inert, don't cause inflammation, and do not "go bad." They have been in use for decades and have a proven track record. Because the implanted lenses are flexible, they fold up very small and can be injected into the eye through a very small incision. Once inside the eye, they unfold like a flower and don't move. You cannot feel the lens in your eye ... your eye will feel normal afterwards.

How will the new implant affect my vision?

The new implant in your eye is optically clear. It should make your vision clearer and reduce glare that was caused by your prior cataract.

How will the new implant affect my eyeglass prescription?

One of the neat things about cataract surgery is that we can change the overall prescription of your eye. The new implant comes in different prescriptions, just like glasses or contact lenses. The power of the implant will determine if you are nearsighted or farsighted.

Most people prefer to have clear distance vision, and choose an implant that will allow them to see far-away objects like the television or road signs. If you have extremely thick glasses now, you'll be pleased to learn that after your cataract surgery you'll be less dependent upon them. You <u>may</u> be able to see at distance without any glasses at all! We will be measuring your eyes before surgery to pick the correct implant prescription power for you.

Why do I need my eyes "measured?"

We need to measure your eyes ahead of time to pick the correct lens implant to put into your eye. When we perform cataract surgery, we remove the cataract from your eye … but it has to be replaced with a new lens in order for you to see afterwards. The new plastic implant is a magnifying glass, and just like glasses or contact lenses, the implant comes in different prescriptions.

Now, it's pretty easy to measure you for eyeglasses. We use an eye chart in the office and can spend all day holding up different lenses in front of you, tweaking your vision to perfection.

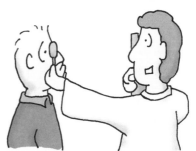

We can't do this trial-and-error approach in the middle of your surgery. We can't tape an eye chart on the operating room ceiling and swap implants in and out of your eye ... all the time asking you "what's clearer ... one or two?" It's just not feasible! Instead, we calculate what lens you'll need AHEAD of time.

How do you calculate my implant power?

We calculate the power of your new implant using two measurements: the length of your eye and the steepness of your cornea. We take these measurements, and using special mathematical formulas, determine the correct implant lens for you.

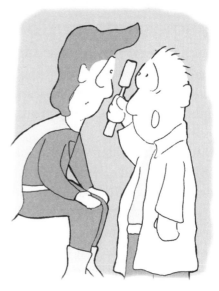

"It's just as we suspected, Super Man. You have "optic nerves of steel."

In other words, we compare YOUR eye measurements to the eye measurements of ten thousand OTHER PEOPLE with similar eyes and say to ourselves:

> "The implant power that gave the majority of THOSE people good vision will, hopefully, be the same implant power that gives YOU good distance vision as well!"

This tends to work well on average. However, your eyes might not be "average." As individuals, we have unique ocular anatomy. Sometimes, people end up a little more near- or farsighted than we predicted. This is correctable with glasses/contacts, but some people are a little disappointed that they still require glasses for best vision.

Fortunately, most people end up with good vision and are able to see well at distance with little or no glasses required. You might still need eyeglasses for "perfect" (20/20) vision, however.

I wear contact lenses now … is this going to affect my measurements?

You should stop wearing your contacts a few weeks before we measure your eyes. Contact lenses can distort our measurements and make our implant calculation inaccurate. This is especially true with hard contact lenses. Let us know if you wear contacts.

I've had LASIK in the past. Is this going to affect my cataract surgery?

Prior LASIK will not affect your surgery, but will make it harder to predict your eyeglass prescription afterwards.

When you had LASIK, the corneal surface of your eye was reshaped with a laser. The implant calculations we use can't take into account your prior operations unless we know what your prior refractive error was. We don't know how much laser energy was used. We don't know the size of the treatment zone ablated. These unknowns make it more challenging to pick the "correct" implant power to put back into your eye.

It can be helpful to obtain your LASIK records to see what your prior measurements were, and our surgical coordinator will help with this. Unfortunately, many people had their LASIK years ago by another doctor. If your laser surgery was more than seven years ago, these records may no longer exist! Many paper-based charts are incinerated after seven years to save space!

Don't worry, we can still calculate your lens implant power and you'll likely have good distance vision after surgery. However, the "unpredictability" is a little bit higher and there is an even greater chance that you'll need some glasses for crisp distance vision. This is important for you to know, as most people who had LASIK are motivated to be "eyeglass free." We want you to be prepared and not angry if you end up in glasses again.

If my prescription is off, can you swap out my implant?

There is risk with surgery, and we want to avoid another operation. However, if your prescription ends up WAY different then expected, and LASIK correction doesn't appeal to you, then a lens exchange may sometimes be an option.

But wait ... isn't the goal of cataract surgery to get me out of glasses?

The goal of cataract surgery is to reduce glare and make your vision crisper, NOT to get you out of glasses. While it is wonderful if you end up less reliant on glasses ... this is a benefit, and not the main reason for this operation.

After surgery, many people have good enough distance vision to drive without glasses ... but perfect 20/20 distance vision is not always possible without a little help from spectacles. Also, you will definitely need some kind of reading glass or bifocal.

There are some new "premium implants" on the market which may make your end-prescription MORE predictable, but even with these new implants there is no guarantee you'll be without some kind of correction. We'll discuss these premium implants in the next chapter.

Why would LASIK give a more predictable prescription than cataract surgery?

With LASIK, a laser beam is used to reshape the surface of the cornea on the OUTSIDE of the eye to change your prescription. This outer ocular surface is easier to measure and manipulate with a laser beam and the end refractive results are quite predictable.

With cataract surgery, however, we are replacing the lens INSIDE the eye. The interior anatomy of the eye is different for everyone. It is impossible to predict 100 percent what prescription (if any) you'll need after this type of surgery.

Can you just give me monovision so I won't need reading glasses?

Monovision is when one eye is set for distance, while the other is set for near. Many contact lens wearers use a "monovision contact prescription" to avoid reading glasses. Most will set their dominant eye for distance and their non-dominant eye set for reading.

While some people tolerate this imbalance well, other people hate monovision. The disparity between their eyes makes them sick to their stomach and unsteady on their feet. The blur at distance ruins their depth perception for driving, and reading becomes a chore because one eye is doing all the work.

Imagine if we set your eyes permanently this way during your surgery. If you don't like your monovision, it's going to be hard to change those implants! At least with glasses or contacts we can take them off or pop them out.

If you've been using monovision contacts for years without issue (or your eyes are "naturally" focused this way), then we may purposefully shoot for monovision after discussing this during your clinic visit.

In the end, most people prefer to have both eyes in synch with each other. You can always put a contact in one eye for monovision afterwards if you really want it.

Can you purposefully make me nearsighted so I can read without glasses?

Most people prefer to have good distance vision and cataract surgery is an opportunity to set your eye's focus for that. However, some nearsighted people are able to read without any glasses at all.

These people read all day long and can't tolerate reading glasses at all ... but don't seem to mind glasses for watching television or driving!

If you are one of these nearsighted creatures, we can purposefully leave you nearsighted to maintain your current focus. It's important you tell us about your post-operative "visual goals" to help make this decision.

I only have a cataract in one of my eyes. How might this affect my prescription goals?

When choosing your implant, we have to keep your ocular balance in mind. We don't want to make your eyes too "different" from each other or you will be uncomfortable afterwards. If we make you nearsighted in one eye while your non-operated eye remains farsighted, your glasses will end up lopsided and the resulting image disparity will give you eye-strain and headaches. Your brain won't like it!

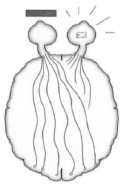

In these cases, we may purposefully under-correct you to give you better "balance." You'll still be in glasses, but at least you'll be comfortable. We will, of course, discuss this with you prior to surgery.

Chapter 3
❧ Premium Implants ❧

Tomoka "Eye-Toons"

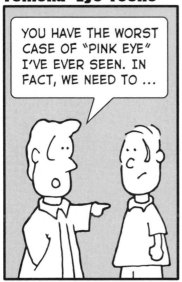

YOU HAVE THE WORST CASE OF "PINK EYE" I'VE EVER SEEN. IN FACT, WE NEED TO ...

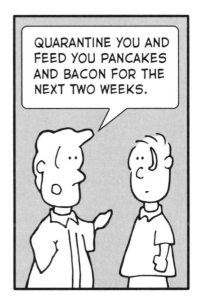

QUARANTINE YOU AND FEED YOU PANCAKES AND BACON FOR THE NEXT TWO WEEKS.

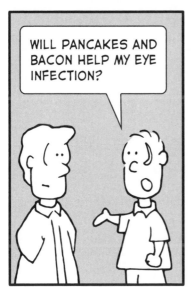

WILL PANCAKES AND BACON HELP MY EYE INFECTION?

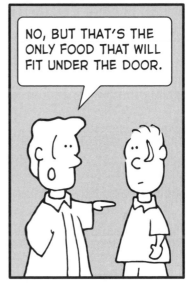

NO, BUT THAT'S THE ONLY FOOD THAT WILL FIT UNDER THE DOOR.

Premium Implants

They might give you better results

Implant technology has improved over the past decade and there are now several "premium" implants on the market that can decrease your dependence on glasses.

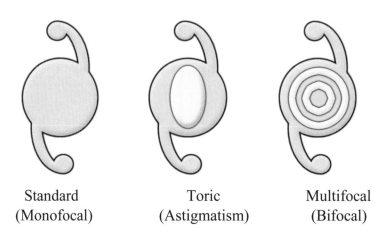

Standard	Toric	Multifocal
(Monofocal)	(Astigmatism)	(Bifocal)

What are my lens implant options?

While most people choose a "regular" implant for their eye, there are a couple of advanced implants on the market. Depending upon your visual goals (and also your personal eye measurements) you may have a better result with one of these "premium" implants.

Let's review the different types of implant we currently use:

Standard Lens Implant
This implant is utilized with most of our patients and has been in use and refined over decades. It allows great vision, is highly stable, and has excellent clarity. The only downsides are that it doesn't fix astigmatism (if you have any) and it is only in focus for far distances ... in other words, you'll definitely need glasses to read.

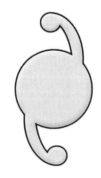

This lens is very good and what most people choose. As long as you don't mind wearing readers or bifocals (and don't have much astigmatism) this is probably the correct lens for you. Plus, this is the lens implant that your medical insurance pays for, so this works out nicely!

Toric (Astigmatism) Implant

If you have significant astigmatism, then a Toric implant is a better choice. A Toric implant counteracts your eye's natural astigmatism and tends to give you a better end prescription after surgery. You'll still need readers/bifocals, but your distance vision will be clearer and there's a much better chance you'll have good distance vision without eyeglass correction.

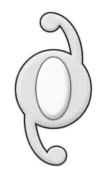

Toric lenses are a really great technology without much downside. The only reason EVERYONE with astigmatism doesn't use these implants is because medical insurance will not cover the additional cost of this lens (though insurance still pays for the surgery itself).

When we measure your eyes, we can tell if you have any astigmatism, and let you know whether a Toric lens is a good option. After all, if you don't HAVE astigmatism, there's no point using this implant!

Multifocal

This lens is neat because it has a dual lens built in. This means you can see both distance and near! If you are active, and your goal is to get out of glasses entirely, then this may be the right implant for you. While these multifocal lenses work, there are a couple of downsides. One is cost … like the Toric lens, insurance does not cover the additional cost of the lens itself.

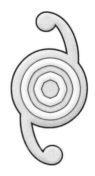

Another is decreased contrast sensitivity. In other words, "whites aren't as white and darks aren't as dark." Most people quickly adapt and don't notice any contrast change. If you have any pre-existing eye problems like macular degeneration or diabetic retinopathy, then this becomes more problematic.

Some people notice small ring-shaped halos around lights at night. Admittedly, most people with cataracts were ALREADY experiencing halos (such that small rings might actually be a huge improvement). However, these halos can really annoy some people.

If you have a visually demanding job or discriminating personality, this type of lens might be a poor choice. If you are a pilot, engineer, or you find yourself constantly cleaning smudges on your glasses ... a multifocal implant may not be the best option.

Most people are extremely happy with their Multifocal lens - but it's important to discuss your goals and expectations with this type of implant.

Why doesn't my insurance pay for the "premium lenses?"

The premium lens implants aren't covered by medical insurance as they are considered cosmetic (just like LASIK laser surgery is considered cosmetic). All other surgical charges incurred with these lenses ARE covered just the same as when the "standard" implants are used.

What is astigmatism?

The surface of the cornea (the clear window that makes up the front of your eye) is normally spherical and round like a basketball. With astigmatism, however, the cornea is shaped more like a football. It is steeper along one axis, and flatter along another.

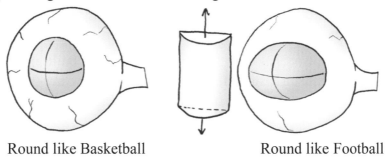

Round like Basketball   Round like Football

We all have a little astigmatism ... but some people have a lot, and this can affect both your glasses prescription and change your implant options.

How do you fix astigmatism using glasses and contacts?

Astigmatism is very easy to fix with glasses. When we make your glasses, we grind the "mirror image" of your football into the glass itself, and rotate the lenses in your frames so that the footballs "cancel" each other out. This gives you very clear vision (though it can make your glasses thick and cause distortion at the edge of your frames).

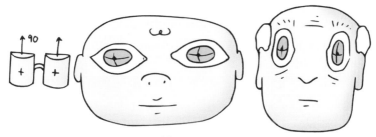

Astigmatism can occur at different angles and change as we age.

We can also fix astigmatism with contact lenses, but this is harder. We can melt the correcting football into the front of a contact lens (this is called a "toric contact") but contacts have a tendency to spin on the surface of the eyeball. Every time you blink, your contact can rotate, and the footballs go "off axis" from each other. This gives you intermittent blurry vision as that contact spins around all day.

How do the "premium" Toric implants fix my astigmatism?

The Toric implant has the "football" correction built in. After injecting this implant inside the eye, we rotate the toric implant around a 360-degree axis until the "football" has lined up perfectly to counteract your eye's "football."

This results in a much better (and more predictable) refractive result. You still might need some glasses for the best distance vision, but you'll be a lot less dependent on them.

How can you tell if I'm a good Toric implant candidate?

During your office visit, we will discuss your lens implant options. While we bring up the possibility, we don't always go into great detail about the Toric implants. At this point in our conversation, most people feel so overwhelmed by the prospect of cataract surgery that an extended discussion of astigmatism and footballs just confuses the issue.

If your current glasses have a large astigmatism correction in them already, then this is a clue that you might need a Toric. However, we won't know until we take your eye measurements during your pre-operative workup.

If your measurements reveal significant corneal astigmatism, then we can talk more about whether a Toric implant would be a good option in your particular case.

What kind of implant do you think I should have?

It really depends upon your visual needs, your measured astigmatism, and if you have any pre-existing eye disease. It usually breaks down to these three choices:

1. If you want to see clearly and don't mind glasses ... a standard implant is great!

2. If you have astigmatism and want to be less dependent on glasses ... a Toric implant may be better.

3. If you hate being dependent on glasses (including reading glasses) and have healthy eyes, no astigmatism, and no "obsessive-compulsive" tendencies ... a Multifocal implant might be wonderful!

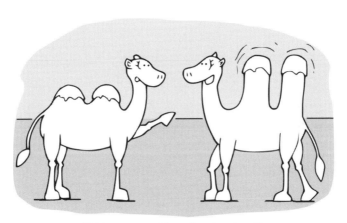

Did you get implants, too?

Chapter 4

Laser Cataract Surgery

Tomoka "Eye-Toons"

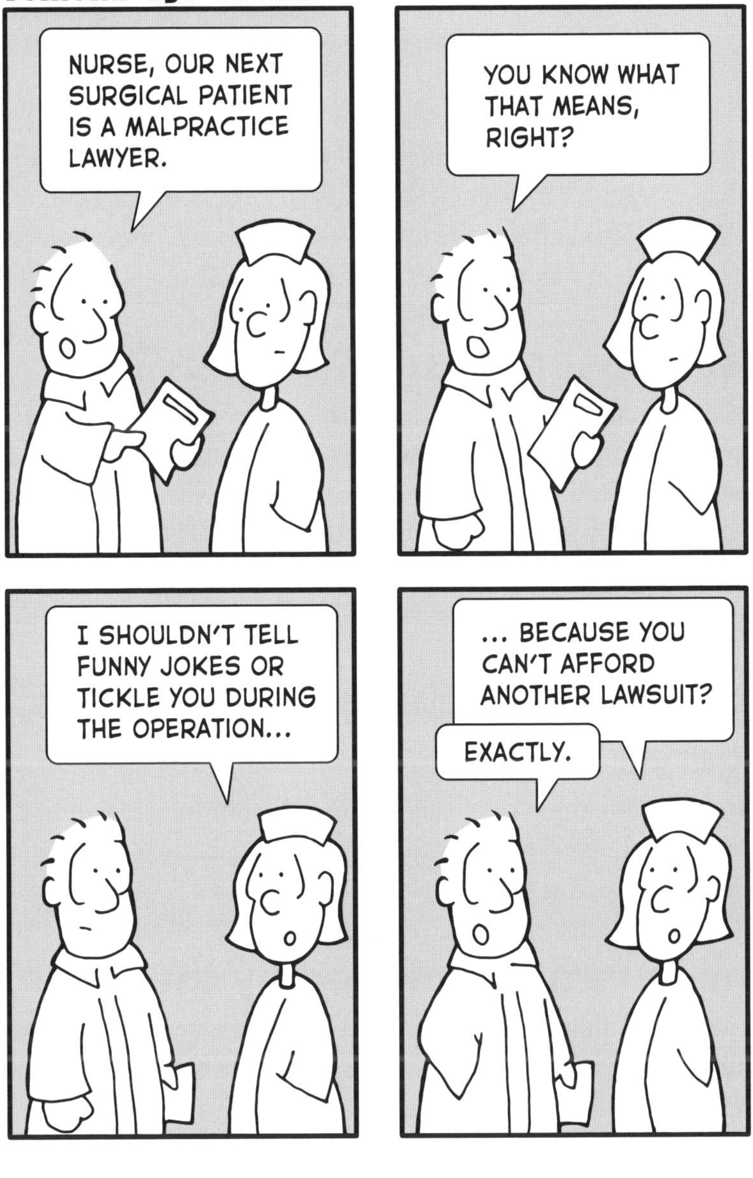
NURSE, OUR NEXT SURGICAL PATIENT IS A MALPRACTICE LAWYER.
YOU KNOW WHAT THAT MEANS, RIGHT?
I SHOULDN'T TELL FUNNY JOKES OR TICKLE YOU DURING THE OPERATION...
... BECAUSE YOU CAN'T AFFORD ANOTHER LAWSUIT?
EXACTLY.

Laser Cataract Surgery

Cataract surgery is a highly developed operation that has undergone many improvements over the years. Ultrasonic phacoemulsification, viscoelastic gels, and premium implant technologies have improved surgical technique and decreased operative risk. Today, cataract surgery is the most common surgical procedure performed across America.

Laser cataract surgery is the newest advancement in this field. With "bladeless surgery," a laser beam is used to perform several steps of the operation. This refinement improves the overall "precision" of your surgery and may make your operation safer and more predictable.

What is laser cataract surgery?

With laser cataract surgery, several steps of the operation are performed using a precision laser and sophisticated computer tracking. The initial corneal incisions are constructed with the laser and the cataract is actually "broken up" using the laser. The laser can be used to make precise cuts in the peripheral cornea to minimize astigmatism. This makes the operation safer and improves your vision afterwards.

Is this the same thing as "bladeless" surgery?

Yes. Instead of using a steel scalpel to make our incisions into the eye, we use the laser. This allows more control and decreases the chance of a wound leak afterwards.

Is the cataract removed by the laser?

While the laser helps us "break" the cataract apart, the laser doesn't actually "remove" the lens itself. The operation still involves entering the eye and manually removing the cataract fragments using a vacuum (phacoemulsification). The overall process of cataract surgery is largely unchanged - the cloudy cataract is still removed and replaced with a clear lens implant.

What are the benefits to having laser?

There are several benefits to laser surgery:

1. The main incisions into the eye are created in a "bladeless" fashion. These incisions are easier to place and their precise construction results in less "wound leakage" afterwards.

2. Small amounts of astigmatism are easier to fix as the laser can create "relaxing incisions" to minimize corneal distortion.

3. The capsulorhexis (the round hole created in the front part of the cataract) is created with the laser. This leads to decreased intra-operative risk and potentially better alignment of the implant inside your eye.

4. The laser helps to break up the cataract itself, leading to less phacoemulsification energy needed inside your eye. This means less trauma and potentially a quicker healing time after surgery.

Why are you using the laser now?

We take great satisfaction in being on the forefront of new technology, but not at the risk of "experimenting" with your eyes with unproven technology. The first generation of cataract laser had limitations. We wanted to make sure the kinks were "worked out" before bringing this technology to our community. The latest generation of lasers have a proven track record of good results so we are now offering this advancement to our patients.

Will the laser fix my astigmatism?

The laser can also eliminate astigmatism by reshaping the corneal surface with precisely placed corneal incisions. The laser, combined with the Toric implant, allows us to treat a wide range of astigmatism and do so more precisely than in the past. This further decreases your dependence on glasses after surgery.

How is "cataract laser" different than LASIK?

LASIK surgery involves sculpting and resurfacing the corneal surface of your eyeball in order to improve your visual focus. Whereas the cataract laser passes harmlessly through the cornea and creates incisions on the cataract itself that helps break it up.

Will I still need glasses after laser-assisted cataract surgery?

Laser assisted surgery is a more precise way to perform your operation. The laser helps to minimize your astigmatism and make your end results more predictable. The laser will decrease the likelihood that you'll need glasses afterwards, but there is still no way to guarantee you'll be completely glasses free. We choose your implant's "strength" based upon sophisticated calculations. However, everyone's internal eye anatomy is different and no calculation can compensate for these individual variations. Even with a "perfect" laser-assisted procedure, there is still the possibility that you will need glasses for the best vision.

Will laser surgery fix my near vision?

Cataract laser won't fix your near vision. The standard and Toric implants we use are designed to be "mono-focal" and are usually set for distance vision. If you want to have good near vision as well, the "multi-focal" lens may be an option.

What will the laser feel like during my actual surgery?

Normally, cataract surgery takes about 10-15 minutes to perform. The laser will make the surgery take a little longer as it requires a few minutes to setup. We will numb your eye with drops so you won't feel anything. To apply the laser, a docking "gadget" is gently placed onto your eye. This does not hurt, though you may feel mild pressure. During the laser application, you won't feel anything but your vision will become blurry. We will talk you through this entire process. After the laser is applied, we remove the laser assembly and proceed with your cataract procedure. Don't worry about feeling nervous during any of these steps - we will give you plenty of numbing medicine and can give you more relaxing medicine via your IV if you need it.

Am I a good candidate for laser?

Most people are good candidates for laser cataract surgery. There are a few exceptions, such as people with small pupils, small eyes, corneal opacities, and certain types of glaucoma. Every eye is different, so we'll talk about the relative benefits for you during your consultation and when you come in for your pre-operative measurements.

Why does laser cataract cost more?

Medicare (and most insurance plans) cover the cost of your cataract surgery, which includes the procedure and post-operative visits. However, laser surgery (and premium implants) are not covered. We have attractive financing plans, however, to minimize any financial burden.

This is overwhelming. Can you list my surgical options again?

At this point, you may find yourself overwhelmed with options. Modern technology has given us many lens choices (standard, Toric, Multifocal), and now we have added laser cataract surgery! With this many options, it may be hard to decide what procedure is correct for your eyes. Generally speaking, you'll fall into one of these four categories:

1. Manual Surgery with a Standard Lens

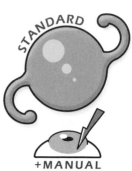

This is the traditional cataract surgery using the standard single-vision lens implant that is covered by your medical insurance. Traditional cataract surgery has an excellent track record and Tomoka Eye has decades of experience with this procedure. Your vision should be much improved after standard surgery, though there is a good chance that you will still need glasses for perfect distance vision. You will definitely need bifocals for close-up work.

2. Laser Surgery with a Standard Lens

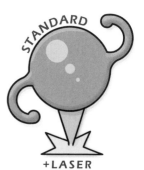

This upgrade utilizes the cataract laser to assist with your operation. This is an excellent choice for people who have small amounts of astigmatism and want to use the latest technology to minimize complications and maximize results. You may still need glasses for distance, but your uncorrected "glasses-free" vision will likely be better than otherwise. You'll still need a bifocal or reading glasses for close-up work.

3. Laser Surgery with a Toric Lens

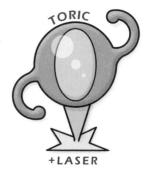

For people with moderate or large amounts of astigmatism, this is the best option. The Toric implant is capable of eliminating massive amounts of astigmatism and this drastically decreases your dependence on glasses after your operation. You may still need glasses afterwards, but they will be much thinner and more comfortable than what you'd end up with otherwise. The Toric implant is a wonderful lens technology and the laser makes this implant work even better. You'll still need glasses for reading.

4. Laser Surgery with a Multifocal Lens

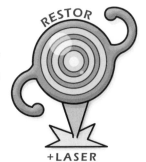

If your goal is to become less dependent on glasses overall, the multi-focal implant may be the best option. This implant has concentric rings built in that help you focus on both distance and near objects. We always use the laser when inserting this lens as it helps to eliminate residual astigmatism, and the laser helps us center the lens in its proper place inside the eye. The multifocal isn't for everyone, but laser-assisted surgery is making this option even more predictable than in the past.

No matter what you choose for your cataract surgery, chances are that you will have a great result. We wouldn't recommend cataract surgery if we didn't think it would help your vision. If you have questions about these options, however, make sure we answer any concerns prior to surgery. You deserve to go into your surgery confident that you've made the best choice for your eyes.

TOMOKA EYE'S LASER

We chose the Alcon LenSx laser platform as this is the most capable laser system on the market today. This remarkable tool combines the latest laser technology with sophisticated eye tracking software. The LenSx laser improves several steps of your eye surgery, making your surgery more precise and predictable.

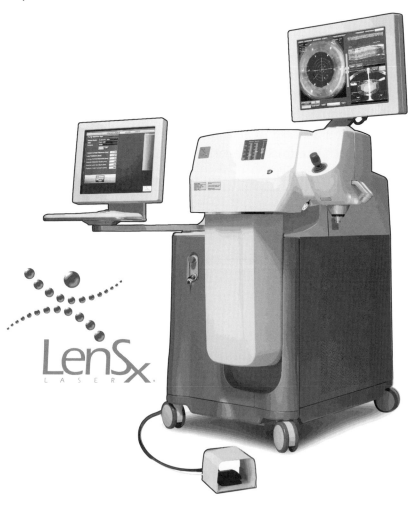

Chapter 5
Setting Up Surgery

Tomoka "Eye-Toons"

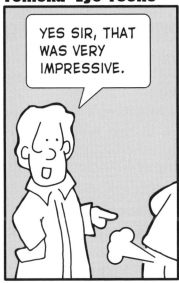

YES SIR, THAT WAS VERY IMPRESSIVE.

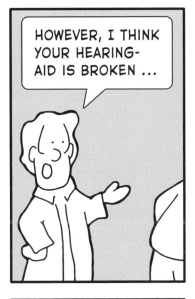

HOWEVER, I THINK YOUR HEARING-AID IS BROKEN ...

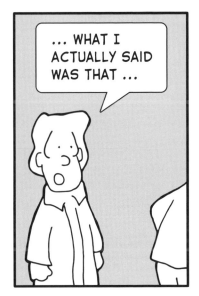

... WHAT I ACTUALLY SAID WAS THAT ...

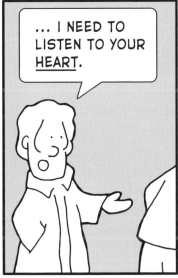

... I NEED TO LISTEN TO YOUR HEART.

Setting up Surgery

Arranging your operation may sound a little daunting, but it's not that bad! Our surgery coordinators will answer any questions and help get everything in order.

What needs to get done before surgery?

Here's what we need to do to arrange your cataract surgery:

1. Speak with our surgery coordinator

We have a dedicated staff member who will give you pre-operative instructions and verify your insurance to help avoid any "financial surprises." Our surgery staff is highly knowledgeable about cataract surgery and can answer any questions.

2. Measurements & paperwork

In order to pick the right lens implant, we need to take your measurements. We can sometimes perform these measurements at the same time as your primary visit, but quite often, we need to set this up on another day when we can provide you with a dedicated technician. These measurements can usually be done without dilating your pupils.

3. Get your drops

You'll be using eye drops before your surgery to decrease the risk of infection and inflammation. You start using these drops three days prior to your surgery date. It is best to have these eye drops filled at your pharmacy ahead of time to avoid last-minute roadblocks. We are closed on the weekend, and you don't want to encounter a problem with your pharmacist.

4. Arrange a driver

You'll need someone to drive you home after surgery, and to bring you to your first post-operative appointment. If this is going to be a problem, our surgery coordinators may be able to arrange transportation.

When do you operate?

Each doctor operates on a different day of the week, so this will depend upon your particular surgeon.

Where is my surgery done?

We perform all surgeries at our surgical center. The Tomoka Surgery Center is located adjacent to our central Ormond Beach office. If you've never been there, it's quite easy to find, away from busy intersections, with ample free parking and no stairs to climb.

Why do you operate in a surgery center and not in a hospital?

We prefer working in our outpatient surgery center because it is pleasant and more convenient for all of us. Your time with us is calmer and less "chaotic" than a hospital where other operations (like hernia repairs, heart surgery, breast implants, etc.) may be going on at the same time. Plus, you don't have to park and negotiate through a giant hospital parking garage.

All of our nurses, technicians, staff, and anesthesiologists specialize in eye care and are better prepared for the specific needs of cataract surgery. This efficiency means your actual operating time will be quicker and less nerve-wracking! Our goal is your safety, and we only perform eye surgery in our sterile operating suites under the supervision of a board-certified anesthesiologist.

What drops will I be on?

You will likely be on three different drops for your surgery.

1. Antibiotic
Antibiotics kill bacteria in the eye and decrease the bacterial load around the eyelashes. This decreases the chance of infection during and after your operation.

2. Non-Steroidal Anti-Inflammatory Drug
The NSAIDS are a class of medication that work like Ibuprofen or Motrin. They decrease inflammation and make the eye feel better. This drop actually diffuses to the back of the eye and decreases the chance of post-operative retinal swelling. This protection is particularly important if you have pre-existing diabetes or retinal problems.

3. Steroid Drop
Nothing works better than a steroid for cooling the eye down after surgery and speeding the healing process. Steroid drops usually come in a larger bottle and you'll be on this for several weeks after surgery.

Don't worry about memorizing this. We will give you a simple instruction sheet (with photographs) of your specific drops along with your other paperwork.

Why do I need to use drops BEFORE surgery?

It sounds strange, but you'll actually start your drops BEFORE surgery! The antibiotic drop will clean the eye and decrease your risk of postoperative infection. The anti-inflammatory drops will speed healing time and decrease your risk of swelling.

These prescription dropper bottles seem rather small. Am I going to run out?

They are small, but should last the required duration. The antibiotic and the NSAID usually come in a tiny bottle (and may be expensive), so be sure to put only a single drop in at a time and try not to miss the eye.

If you find you are missing your eye a lot, you might need assistance from friends or family members to avoid wasting drops. Assuming you apply them properly, you will stop each medication as the bottle runs out.

How long do I use these drops?

You'll start these drops three days before surgery. You'll continue them for several weeks afterward. Most of the time, you simply use the drops until they run out (or we tell you to stop them).

Chapter 6

❧ Maximizing Outcomes ❧

Tomoka "Eye-Toons"

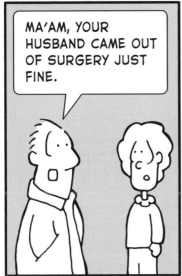

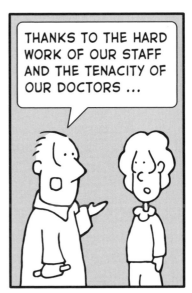

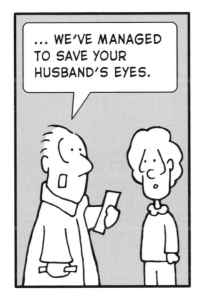

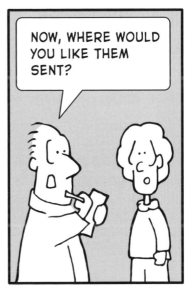

Maximizing Outcomes

Safety precautions for good results

Complications! This is probably the thing that worries you most about having a cataract surgery, right? This is your eye, after all, and the thought of something bad happening to your vision can be terrifying!

Cataract surgery is pretty safe overall. Complications are rare ... but it's only fair to fully disclose what "could happen" with this procedure, and also emphasize the efforts we make in keeping your surgery safe.

Safe, low-risk surgery is one of the reasons we became ophthalmologists. This is a satisfying operation for us because almost everyone is extremely happy with their surgical results.

Is cataract surgery risky?

Cataract surgery is one of the most successful surgeries performed in the United States. About 95% of people have improved vision after this procedure. Most of the remaining 5% already had pre-existing eye disease like macular degeneration or diabetic retinopathy that limited their visual potential.

Despite the overall success, unexpected things can happen. EVERY cataract surgeon has complications because EVERY eye is different. Eyes react differently under the microscope and everyone heals differently.

As ophthalmologists, we work at high volume and this repetition keeps us "fresh and consistent," with lower complication rates than most surgical fields. Even so, we still see occasional problems.

What are potential complications with this surgery?

We discuss complications during your pre-operative appointments, but we'd like to readdress a few here. Cataract surgery, compared to most surgeries, is quite safe with a high success rate. Still, despite all precautions and good intentions, complications can occur.

We do NOT LIKE complications, nor does our surgical team. We are constantly looking for ways to make your surgery safe and uneventful. Here are some steps we take to minimize your risk and maximize your outcome:

Infection – We prescribe antibiotic drops before and after surgery to lessen the bacterial load around your eye and eyelid. We use sterile operating rooms where we perform ONLY ocular surgery (no abdominal surgery or "dirty wound" operations here). We clean the eye before starting your procedure and perform all operations fully "masked and gowned" via strict sterile technique. After your surgery we place an antibiotic in your eye and you'll use more at home. We check your eyes several times during the first week (the most dangerous time for infection) to make sure you're doing well. As you can imagine, our infection rate is very low.

Inflammation – You will be using both a steroid and an NSAID (non-steroid anti-inflammatory) drop after surgery to cool your eye down. During surgery we attempt to minimize the amount of "energy" used to remove your cataract. If your eye has a propensity for inflammation or swelling (such as with diabetes) we prescribe a longer dosage of your NSAID drop to be on the safe side.

Corneal Edema – The cornea usually swells after surgery and this causes blur. This is normal. While this swelling typically resolves within a week, we attempt to minimize this edema by using protective 'gels' during your surgery. We also use minimal energy settings when breaking apart the cataract to minimize vibration damage in the eye.

Retinal Edema – The NSAID anti-inflammatory drop we prescribe for you decreases the risk of post-operative retinal edema. Plus, we check your vision at every exam, and perform retinal scans when you're not seeing as well as expected.

Retinal Detachment – We attempt to minimize unnecessary manipulation during your surgery, and we check you several times after your operation. We also have operators available who answer our phones after hours (even in the middle of the night) and who can contact us at home if you're having odd visual symptoms.

Bleeding – Bleeding in the eye is uncommon, as this surgery is usually "bloodless." If you are on blood thinners and we are planning more extended anesthesia or a lengthy operation, we may stop your blood thinner ahead of time (after obtaining clearance from your primary doctor).

Insufficient Capsular Support – If the supporting capsular bag is not intact (the natural pocket that holds your new implant in place), then it becomes tricky to insert your new lens. In these cases, we clean the eye with a procedure called a "vitrectomy" and may place a different style implant that sits more securely inside your eye. You may require a second surgery to remove the remaining cataract fragments. This extends surgical time and recovery, but gives a better result and the vision is usually fine.

Glaucoma – We check your pressure the day after surgery and use drops if there is a temporary pressure spike. If the pressure is very high, we'll even occasionally "burp" the incision to remove excess fluid from the eye. This is done at your office checkup and is painless.

Refractive Error – Glasses will fix any residual focus issues. In the extremely rare case of high-refractive error (for example, you end up extremely nearsighted) we can perform a lens implant "exchange."

Pain – We use anesthesia via your IV, topically on the surface of your eye, and even INSIDE your eye to minimize discomfort. We have anesthesiologists who monitor and give larger doses of pain medication if required to keep you comfortable.

Anxiety – Most people are nervous about their surgery and may even have claustrophobia. We give you plenty of anti-anxiety medications to calm you and make your surgery safer and more enjoyable.

Fortunately, big complications are rare. Even when there ARE difficulties with your cataract surgery, the end result is usually still great (though the healing time and recovery time might be longer). It is rare that you might actually end up with worse vision ... but it can happen. That's why we wait until your cataract is bad enough so the benefits of your surgery (seeing better) outweigh these potential risks (not seeing better).

What signs might indicate that my surgery could be complicated?

Complications are hard to predict. There are some clues that a surgery is going to be more difficult than average. These include:

- An extremely dense-looking cataract
- Poor pupil dilation
- Prior eye surgery
- Flomax or other urinary medication use
- Extreme near- or farsightedness
- Co-existing eye disease such as Pseudoexfoliation Syndrome or Fuchs' Dystrophy

Why would a dense cataract make surgery difficult?

When we remove your cataract, we don't remove it in one giant piece. Instead, we use a "phacoemulsification machine." This tool vibrates at ultrasonic frequencies and breaks up your cataract into tiny pieces. We then vacuum these pieces out. This decreases your operating time and makes for much faster healing afterwards.

You can think of this vibrating tool like a miniaturized jack-hammer that chips away at your cataract. If your cataract is dense like a rock, then more energy will be required to break it apart. The more energy used, the more swelling after surgery, and the longer the recovery time.

If your cataract is really bad and dense like a "diamond" ... our phaco-machine might not be able to break it apart safely. In these cases, we fall back to the older methods of surgery (extending the surgical excision and removing the remaining cataract in one piece). This dramatically lengthens your surgery time and will require placing stitches in the eye.

Extremely dense cataracts are the major cause of surgical difficulties. This why we recommend addressing your cataracts before they get this bad.

Why does my pupil size matter?

Your cataract/lens is suspended inside your eye immediately behind your iris (the colored part of your eye). The black pupil is a round hole in the middle of your colored iris. To reach your cataract, we need to work THROUGH your pupil to get to the cataract underneath.

When you dilate well, your pupil is very wide, and cataract surgery is easy. We have lots of working room to maneuver instruments and a good view of the entire cataract.

Small pupils are a different matter. A small pupil makes it hard to manipulate the cataract. It's like working through a tiny keyhole. We have less working room and a limited view of how your cataract is doing as we break it apart. This is especially problematic if you have a rock-hard cataract - it is difficult to manipulate a large cataract through a tiny pupil. It's like picking a lock safe on a rocking boat during a hurricane!

How do you handle poorly dilated eyes during surgery?

If your pupil is very small and refuses to dilate, we can still perform a safe surgery, but we'll need to perform extra surgical steps to make your pupil cooperate. This includes:

1. Epinephrine - This is a powerful dilating medication that we can use inside the eye during surgery to coax the pupil larger.

2. Iris Hooks - These look like miniature candy canes. We use them along the periphery of the iris to temporarily stretch the pupil.

3. Malyugin Ring - Similar to iris hooks, this is an expanding spring that holds the pupil and keeps it dilated.

Manipulating the iris during surgery can be irritating to the eye, so we'll give you more pain medication. If, during your clinic visit, it is obvious that you'll need pupil stretching, we will even change your anesthesia method ahead of time to insure you are comfortable.

Why do some people dilate poorly?

Some people have small pupils that do not dilate well despite aggressive use of dilating eye drops. Some of this is genetic and some of this is aging. The iris muscle that controls pupil dilation can atrophy as we age.

What problems does Flomax cause?

Flomax is a common medication used to help urine flow. It works by relaxing smooth muscles throughout the body. While this works great for the urinary tract, this "relaxation" can create challenges during your eye surgery. Flomax and drugs like it cause a condition called "floppy iris syndrome."

What is floppy iris syndrome?

The iris is the colored part of the eye - some people have blue irises and others have brown. The iris is a muscle as well, and this muscle makes your pupil large or small depending upon ambient lighting.

The drug Flomax makes your iris muscle "relax" and become "floppy." This relaxation can be so intense that when we make our initial microincision into the eye, the iris can bulge forward and actually block that incision! This makes surgery challenging, as you can imagine. The iris gets in the way and makes it hard to proceed with your operation without causing irritation to this tissue as we maneuver inside the eye with our instruments.

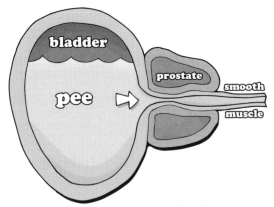

Urinary medications like Flomax are designed to relax smooth muscles.

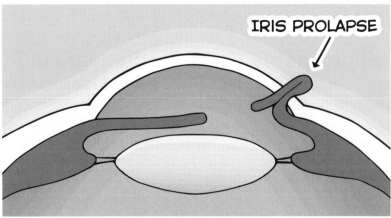

The iris is made of smooth muscle. If this muscle relaxes, it becomes "floppy" and hard to work with.

How do you handle floppy iris syndrome?

There are many modern methods to deal with floppy iris . . . we use the same tools that we use for someone who has poor pupil dilation. We'll use epinephrine at the start of the operation as this medication decreases floppiness. In addition, if the iris is "acting funny" we'll place iris hooks or a Malyugin Ring to hold the iris down in good position.

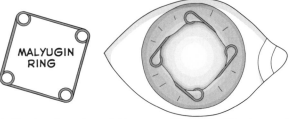

The Malyugin Ring is extremely useful in cases of floppy iris. We also use it for people with poor dilation. This device keeps the pupil dilated during surgery and is very gentle.

If you are on Flomax and have a cataract, we can deal with this ... but there is no doubt that this medication makes cataract surgery difficult. This is especially true if your cataract is extremely dense or you don't dilate well. Floppy iris syndrome is something we see a lot in ophthalmology and the prevalence is increasing (Flomax has gone generic so we're seeing more usage).

I'm already on Flomax ... should I stop it now before surgery?

The effect of this medication on the iris is long-lived, and people can have floppy iris even after a year off the medication. Just be sure to let us know if you are on this medication and you'll be fine.

Can I have floppy iris even if I don't take Flomax?

Yes, some people have a naturally floppy iris muscle that doesn't cooperate during surgery. This is especially true if you have light-colored eyes or pupils that don't dilate well in the office.

What is Pseudoexfoliation Syndrome?

Pseudoexfoliation Syndrome is common, especially if you are of Scandinavian descent. With this condition, a flaky dandruff-like material forms on the surface of your lens/cataract. This material rubs off over a lifetime and can cause glaucoma if the material "clogs the drain" inside your eye.

This material also forms on the support strings that hold your cataract in position behind your iris. These strings are called zonules. These zonular strings surround the cataract/lens in a 360 degree ring, and hold your cataract in place like springs on a trampoline.

With Pseudoexfoliation Syndrome, the flaky material weakens these springs. If the springs break during surgery, the cataract can fall into the back of the eye and will require removal by a retinal surgeon (a second operation).

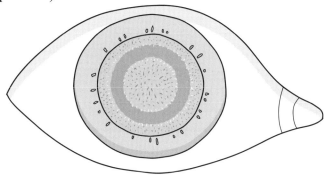

We can detect Pseudoexfoliation Syndrome during a routine eye exam.

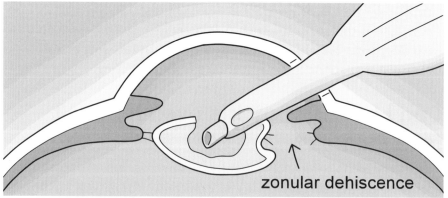

zonular dehiscence

Pseudoexfoliation can weaken the "springs" that hold the cataract in place.

What is Fuchs' Dystrophy?

Fuchs' Dystrophy is a relatively common condition that affects 1-2% of the population. Fuchs' Dystrophy is when the cornea has fewer endothelial pump cells than normal, which puts you at higher risk for corneal decompensation after surgery. That may sound confusing, so let's explain:

The cornea, the clear window that forms the front of your eye, is clear because it is relatively "dehydrated." This may seem odd at first. After all, isn't the eye full of water and covered by tears on the outside? How can the cornea be "dry"?

The cornea is dry because there is a layer of cells on the inner surface of the cornea called endothelial pump cells. These endothelial pump cells continually suck water out of the cornea and pump it back inside the eye. These cellular pumps work like thousands of tiny "bilge pumps" that keep the corneal "ship" dry and afloat.

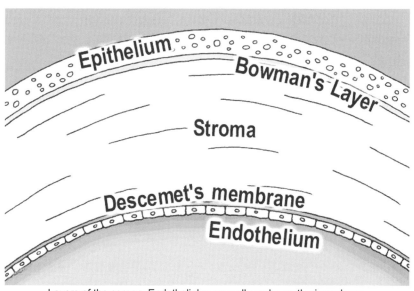

Layers of the cornea. Endothelial pump cells make up the inner layer.

We are all born with a certain number of these pump cells at birth but this number declines with age. You need to maintain a bare minimum of these pumps to keep your cornea dry, and unfortunately, these pump cells don't regenerate when damaged (such as after cataract surgery).

After surgery (even uncomplicated surgery) a percentage of these pump cells stop working and the cornea becomes temporarily "wet" and boggy. This creates blur and halos around lights. Over the next week, this blurriness goes away as the remaining endothelial cells start working again and pump the cornea "dry" again.

People with Fuchs' Dystrophy have less pump cells than the rest of us. After surgery, these corneas take longer to dry because they have so few pump cells left to do the job. Sometimes, there aren't enough pump cells left and the cornea STAYS wet and cloudy. These patients might need a corneal transplant to replace their endothelial cells and make the cornea clear again.

Who is at risk for cornea cloudiness?

The risk of permanent cloudiness is higher with Fuchs', advanced age, and extremely "dense" cataracts. Dense cataracts require more energy to remove and result in more endothelial cell damage and tissue swelling.

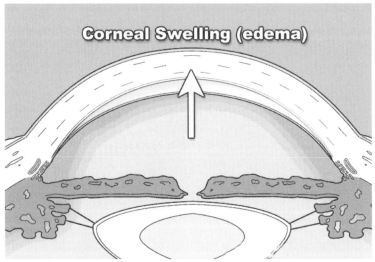

When the cornea swells, it becomes cloudy. This creates blurry vision and patient's often see a "halo" around lights.

If you have these risk factors, and your eye looks like it might have cornea problems after surgery, we'll discuss this prior to surgery.

Most eyes, even with Fuchs' Dystrophy, clear eventually ... but it can sometimes take months and require additional drops.   Corneal repair surgery has improved tremendously, so all is not lost if you end up with a permanently wet cornea. Fortunately, corneal decomposition is rare these days.

What do you do to protect my eye from this cornea damage?

Permanent cloudiness used to be a major problem in the early days of cataract surgery. The older methods of surgery were so aggravating to the endothelium that corneal transplants were common.

Modern surgery is less traumatic to the cornea.   We now use viscoelastic gels to protect the cornea. These gels are injected during surgery to coat the inner surface of the cornea. This gel softens the vibration and heat energy coming from our instruments and keeps the corneal endothelium happy.

I'm extremely nearsighted. How will this affect my surgery?

People who are nearsighted usually have much LONGER and LARGER eyes than usual. A long eye can make your surgery a little challenging as we have to go further into the eye just to get to your cataract. Also, larger eyes are always at higher risk for developing a retinal detachment after surgery.

Despite this, we enjoy performing cataract surgery on nearsighted people as we usually have a lot of "working room" inside the eye, and the prescription improvement after surgery makes these patients extremely happy.

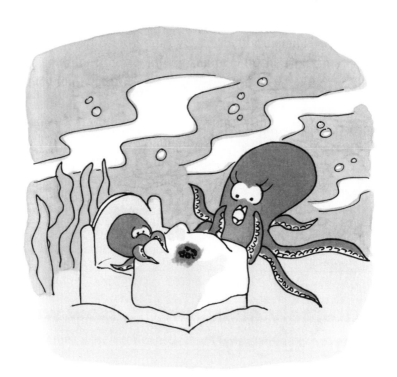

"Oh Timmy, did you ink in your bed again?"

Chapter 7
❧ The Day of Surgery ❧

Tomoka "Eye-Toons"

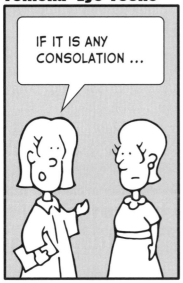

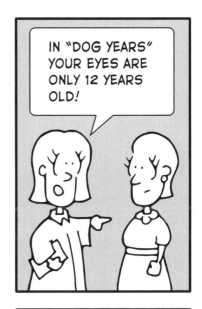

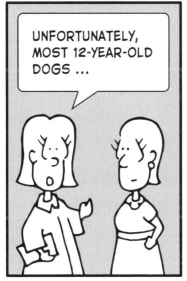

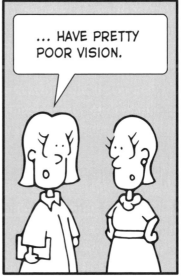

The Day of Surgery

What to expect

The day of surgery is a little stressful for most people. There are a few things you'll need to do before arriving, such as NOT eating, using your medications, and arranging for a driver.

Can I eat breakfast before surgery?

Definitely not! Do not eat or drink anything. You are allowed to drink water with your oral medication, but that's it. Despite the short duration and the minimal anesthesia, this is still a surgery. We give you relaxing medications (sometimes a lot of relaxing medicine if you are anxious) and you will be lying flat. We don't want any food to regurgitate and go down the wrong pipe into your lungs!

Our anesthesiologists are top notch and will take no chances with your health. They are ALSO very strict - if you eat anything, we will cancel surgery and reschedule. Safety is the key here and there is no point in taking unnecessary risks. We want you to have a great outcome!

My cataract isn't scheduled until the afternoon. Can I eat an early snack?

Nope. No exceptions! We'll give you some coffee and a muffin right AFTER your surgery, but don't eat anything prior to surgery. Feel free to eat a hearty meal the evening before, though, as long as it's before midnight. You should avoid coffee or alcohol in the evening, however, as these can promote reflux and heartburn.

I can't wake up without a pick-me-up. Can I have coffee in the morning?

No coffee, no milk, no creamer, nada. Caffeine can cause reflux and creamer is considered food.

If it makes you feel better, we'll have a hearty breakfast and a big cup of coffee the morning of your surgery! Your doctor will eat a delicious breakfast that will give him a clear head and steady hands for your surgery!

What time do I come in?

We'll be calling you the day prior to surgery to tell you what time to arrive (unless you have Monday surgery ... in which case our staff will call you on Thursday). We need you there early enough to get your eye dilated, take care of paperwork, and to place your IV.

Should I bring a driver?

Yes. You need someone to drive you home after surgery. While many of our patients feel fine afterward and see well enough with their other eye to drive, it is NOT a good idea. We give you relaxing medicine during surgery that can make you quite groggy. If transportation is going to be a problem for you, let our surgery coordinator know and we may be able to arrange something for you. The staff won't let you leave if you don't have someone to drive you.

You may also need someone to drive you to your post-operative appointment the next day. This will depend upon your overall binocular vision and your comfort in driving with a newly operated eye that may still be blurry.

What should I bring with me the morning of surgery?

Here are the things you should bring with you:

>**Friend or Family** – Bring someone to help you with paperwork and to drive you home after surgery.

>**Insurance Cards and ID** – Our surgery center may not have this information, so bring your insurance information with you.

Medications – Bring enough of your normal oral medications to sustain you while away from home. Our nurse will discuss this with you.

List of ALL medications – Bring a list of all your prescription medications, including dosage and strength, so our anesthesiologist can review them.

Sweater or jacket – Surgery centers are usually cold, especially when you are waiting. Dress in layers, preferably with loose sleeves to help with your IV placement.

Reading material – Bring busy work or something to read. It can take a while for your eyes to dilate.

What do I tell my driver? Do they have to wait around?

It will take a while for you to dilate. Surgery itself, however, is surprisingly quick. We'll try to give your driver fair warning. It's probably better if they hang around to receive your post-op instructions. Two heads are better than one!

Should I take my normal medications the morning of surgery?

No. Only medications for blood pressure, your heart, or acid reflux inhibitors should be taken, with a SIP of WATER. Our nurse will review your medications and discuss particular medications with you prior to surgery.

I have diabetes. Do I take my insulin or diabetic pills the morning of surgery?

No. Your blood glucose needs to be normal to high the morning of surgery. We can check your blood glucose at the surgery center.

I am on a blood thinner. Do I continue this?

Yes. Cataract surgery is essentially a bloodless procedure, so you can continue all your normal blood thinners like Coumadin, Warfarin, Plavix, or Aspirin.

The only exception to this is when we perform retrobulbar-block anesthesia. If you require one of these "blocks" we will have already discussed this during your pre-operative appointment and will have already gotten clearance to stop your blood thinner prior to surgery.

I'm on oxygen, should I bring it with me?

Yes, you should bring enough with you to last a three-hour stay.

May I wear makeup? Perfume?

Heavens no! Do not wear makeup on the day of surgery. Makeup contains odd chemicals, such as guanine, which is obtained from fish scales. You do NOT want that stuff inside your eye. That means no eyeliner, no mascara … nothing on the face. You'll have to look pretty another day. No perfume is allowed either, for similar reasons.

What do I do with my hair?

Wear your hair loose, with no bands or pins to pull it back. We'll place a hair-cover over your head to contain those locks.

I have a hearing aid. Can I wear this?

Yes, wear this to our office. We may take the hearing aid out during surgery, depending upon what eye is being operated on. You can put it back in afterwards, so you can communicate and hear your post-operative nurses talking to you. Your hearing aid remains on your stretcher in a plastic cup to make sure it isn't misplaced.

What about dentures ... do I need to remove them?

You can leave your dentures in, unless we tell you otherwise.

What kind of clothing should I wear?

You will be wearing your own clothing during this surgery, so wear something loose and comfortable with flat shoes. Dress in layers in case you get cold.

We will be placing an IV in your arm, so you don't want to wear tight sleeves. Also, you'll have a blood-pressure cuff around your upper arm, so wear something with loose enough sleeves so that we can slide this cuff up under your arm. You should not wear constricting sweatshirts or pullovers that are hard to get off.

Do you use an anesthesiologist? Do you need one?

We have board-certified anesthesiologists working with us. Most surgeries are quick and require minimal anesthesia. Still, it's nice knowing you have an experienced person there who can monitor you carefully to insure a good outcome and keep you comfortable.

Will you put me to sleep during my operation?

No. Cataract surgery doesn't take very long and it is better to keep you awake during surgery. However, if you are nervous or anxious, we can monitor you closely and put you into a groggy "twilight sleep" to get you through the case.

No, seriously, I HAVE to be put to sleep if you want to operate near my eye!

On rare occasions, we can perform cataract surgery under "general" anesthesia. This is usually in cases of dementia, agitation, or extreme claustrophobia. However, we can only do general anesthesia if you are healthy. If you have medical problems like heart or lung disease, then it is better to perform general anesthesia in a hospital setting in case of complications from anesthesia itself. If you need general anesthesia, we will need a current EKG, bloodwork, and clearance from your primary doctor. Our surgery coordinators can arrange this.

What will I experience when I come to the surgery center?

Our surgery center is located adjacent to our central Ormond Beach office. In fact, the front door is only a few feet from our lobby entrance.

When you walk inside, you'll be greeted by our front-desk staff who will check you in and help you fill out paperwork. Once everything is in order, we'll bring you back into our pre-operative "checkup" station. Here we recheck your vital signs and recheck your overall health.

We then set you up in a comfortable stretcher bed so you can relax as our experienced nurse puts dilating drops in your eye and places an IV in your arm. Our nurses are all top-notch with many years of experience, so you won't be getting a "student" fumbling with your IV.

You'll have an identification band placed on your wrist and you'll be asked to identify yourself constantly. This will get annoying, but this is a safety precaution to make sure we are doing the correct surgery on the correct person. We even use a marker to identify which eye (right versus left) you are having done. Safety first!

After your drops and IV are in, you can relax until it's your turn. You'll see other patients coming out of surgery ... and you'll see they also look fine and completely relaxed.

What will I experience during the surgery itself?

When it is time for your cataract surgery, you are wheeled back to the operating suite and the operating nurses make sure you are comfortable on the stretcher. This usually involves blankets and positioning of your head and back so that you aren't cold and you feel comfortable. The nurse then cleans the skin around your eye using gauze and cotton swabs. The cleaning solution feels a little cold, but it doesn't sting.

The scrub nurse then drapes a sterile sheet over your head to isolate the eye and keep everything clean and sterile. This drape is a little funny, as your eye will be open while we drape it over you. We'll explain everything we're doing.

Don't worry about being covered either - you won't feel claustrophobic. We position a hose under the drape to give you lots of breathing space and we pump in refreshing air for you to inhale. Plus, we'll be talking to you, playing music, and making sure you feel relaxed.

The surgery itself is pretty straightforward. The doctor will be sitting next to your head, talking to you. There will be a bright light from the microscope. You can't see or feel any instruments, just the doctor's hands resting on your cheek and forehead. You will hear some funny sounds, similar to a vibrating cellular phone, and you'll also hear your doctor talking to the scrub nurse.

Occasionally, you'll feel a little eye pressure. We talk to you during the operation and give you warning before any little pressure changes so you aren't caught unaware. We give you pain medications topically, internally, and through your IV - most people blast through this procedure without much irritation at all!

The surgery itself takes about 15 minutes. Some people are so relaxed that they fall asleep halfway through. We'd prefer if you stay awake, though. We don't like people waking and moving suddenly . . . but sometimes, if everything is going smoothly, we'll let you drift off.

When we are done, we remove the drape and we place antibiotic eye drops in your eye. We then tape a clear shield over the eye and wheel you back out to the post-operative area.

What will I experience in the post-operative area?

The post-operative area is where we sit you up and make sure you are feeling well before we send you home. Here, we'll check your vital signs and make sure you truly feel okay. We give you coffee, juice, or tea and a snack.

After a few minutes, we'll sit you up in a chair and call in friends or family to sit with you. Here, we'll go over your post-operative instructions again.

Once you are feeling collected (and we've answered any last minute questions you might have), you can go home. We'll assist you to your car (and can provide a wheelchair if you need one). Vehicles can be pulled very close to the side of the building.

What extra steps do you take to make surgery safe?

In order to protect you and give you the best results possible, our team constantly monitors and updates our facilities. For example:

- We use board-certified anesthesiologists.
- We run two separate operating suites in order to have redundancy in case of equipment issues.
- We have a generator in case of power outages.
- We attach identification bracelets and constantly recheck to make sure we have the correct person, the correct eye, correct lens implant, etc..
- We stock a backup implant for your case.
- Our facility is checked and accredited for safety and sterility.

Does it hurt?

Cataract surgery doesn't hurt ... we know, as we ask our patients how they are feeling throughout this procedure and we get lots of feedback during post-op appointments. There are a couple of steps when the eye can "sting a little," such as when we drop anesthetic drops on the eye. You may even feel a little pressure during certain steps . . . but pain? Not really.

If the eye is hurting at all, we simply give more anesthetic topically and our anesthesiologist gives more medicine through your IV. We try to keep you comfortable and make the entire experience as stress-free as possible for you.

How much time will surgery take?

The actual cataract surgery itself takes only about 15 minutes. However, it takes quite a bit more time for everything else . . . to get you checked in, IV placed, waiting your turn, preparing the OR, etc. After the surgery, we place drops, remove the IV, and make sure you are feeling OK before leaving. You should plan on about two hours total time in the surgery center.

Will I be able to see the surgical instruments during the operation?

No. You won't see any instruments. You may see a couple of bright lights from the microscope, and some shadows while we work. Many people see funny, colored lights during their operation which brings back memories of the '60s.

I am very nervous about this.

The idea of eye surgery is rather daunting. What if something goes wrong? What if I move during the procedure? I might never see again! These are the thoughts that may be racing through your mind.

Even though this is a novel experience for you, we do this all the time and we'll take good care of you. We will also give you lots of anti-anxiety medicine to keep you relaxed. You'll be relieved when it's all over and we think you'll be surprised by how low stress the actual experience ended up being.

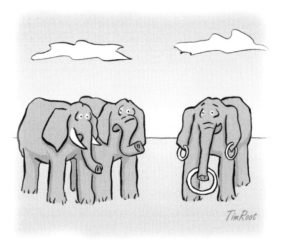

"The earrings were daring,
but that nose ring is too much."

Chapter 8
❧ After Surgery ❧

Tomoka "Eye-Toons"

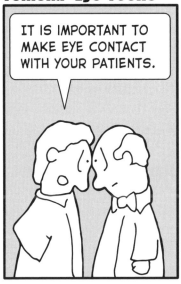

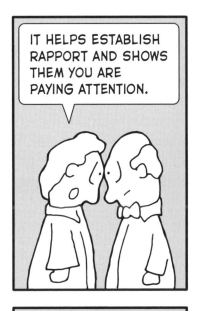

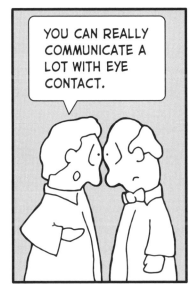

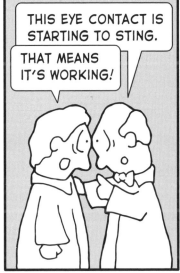

After Surgery

What to expect after your operation

Congratulations, you just had a successful cataract surgery! Most people are so relieved after their operation that they look forward to getting home and resting. Once home, however, you may start having questions about your operated eye!

Will my eye hurt after surgery?

It's rare to actually have pain after surgery, but most people have some irritation. This can be a foreign body sensation or an itchiness to the eye. Many people tell us that it feels like there is a piece of sand or an eyelash stuck in the eye for the first 24 hours afterwards.

Hey, my eye aches a little!

Don't worry. This pain should pass pretty quickly. You can take a pain reliever like Tylenol if you need it. If you are having extreme pain, however, call us!

My eye stings when I put the eye drops in.

Your eye is pretty sensitive and a few of the eye drops you are using can irritate the corneal surface. This sting is normal and should get better in a few days. Continue using your drops . . . they are not damaging the eye.

What should I do when I get home after surgery?

You should probably take it easy. You just had surgery ... and while the operated area is pretty small, the emotional stress may have you pretty zonked. Plus, all the medication we pumped into you can make you groggy. Many people take a nap during the early afternoon. The only real precaution here is to wear that eye shield so that you don't rub the eye unconsciously while you are sleeping.

What kind of vision should I expect?

Your vision is going to be blurry. While you may know people who had "perfect vision" immediately after their surgery, this is the exception, not the rule. Your eye is still dilated from the procedure and your cornea is swollen, so you're not going to be seeing well for a few days. You might even see halos or rings around lights. This is normal.

How long is my vision going to be blurry?

Blurry vision after surgery is normal, especially during the first week or two. This blurriness occurs because the cornea is swollen after your operation. This is a normal response to surgery - ALL tissues in the body become swollen when you perform surgery on them!

The cornea is normally a clear "window" into the eye … and when it becomes swollen, it becomes cloudy and hazy. This makes your vision blurry and seem as if you are looking through cloudy or fogged-up glasses.

Most of this cloudiness will resolve during the first week as the cornea clears, but some people take longer to heal . . . especially if your cataract was dense. As your cornea heals your vision will get better, and you'll become happier with your visual improvement.

I was told to cover my eye. How come?

The number one rule after cataract surgery is:

DON'T RUB THE EYE

We perform this surgery through a self-sealing corneal incision. While that incision has great integrity, we don't want you to rub the eye and cause the incision to leak. This might slow down healing or even increase the chance of infection. So, we send you home with a clear plastic shield to tape over the eye before you sleep. This keeps you from rubbing the eye unconsciously while you snooze.

Many people wear the clear shield home the day of surgery and keep it on that day as a reminder to leave the eye alone. In addition, we put sunglasses in your kit so that you can wear them while walking around outside.

How long will I be wearing this eye shield?

Use the shield for five nights and also when you take naps. This shield will keep you from accidentally rubbing the eye while you are sleeping. Tape the shield over the eye like a pirate patch when you go to bed.

After five nights, your eye will have healed to the point that you can go without the shield. You'll be ready to stop by this point anyway - the tape leaves behind a sticky residue on the skin that is difficult to remove.

Do I have to wear the sunglasses?

No. Sunglasses are optional. We recommend sunglasses the first few days, however, as your eyes may be sensitive to bright sunlight. Also, sunglasses serve as a reminder to not rub your eye if it is feeling irritated.

If the sunglasses are bothering you, or you are fashion conscious, you don't have to wear them . . . just make sure nothing gets in your eye. Don't let pets or children poke you in the eye.

My eye is still dilated. Is this normal?

Yes, the dilating drops we use with surgery tend to last much longer than those in our office. Some people have a dilated eye for days.

When do I come back for my follow-up appointment?

We'll be seeing you back the day after surgery. In addition, we check you at one week, and then a few weeks after that for your final exam and glasses prescription. This would break down to:

Day 1: Surgery
Day 2: Next day checkup
Day 7: One week checkup
Day 21: Final exam and glasses refraction

If you are having BOTH eyes done, we combine appointments to minimize unnecessary visits.

How soon can I have my second cataract surgery?

We often perform your second surgery about two weeks after your first cataract operation. This gives your first eye time to heal and will make it easier to see after your second surgery.

On rare occasions, we'll perform your next surgery after only a week. If the healing is sluggish (or your vision is blurrier than you expected) we can push back the surgery date on your second eye until you are happy with the first.

Can't you just do both eyes at the same time?

No … cataract surgery is trickier than other types of elective surgery (LASIK for example) and everyone heals at a different rate. We want to make sure your first eye is doing great before booking your second eye. It's all about minimizing risk. Some people have a significant amount of blurriness after surgery as well, and you'll have a hard time if BOTH eyes are blurry at the same time.

Do I see you for my follow-up?

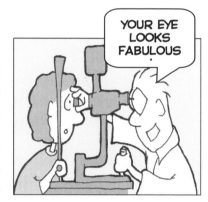

Yes. However, each of our doctors performs surgery on a different morning and sees patients at several offices. The day after surgery, your surgeon may be working at a distant office. It may be more convenient for you to see one of our OTHER doctors for some post-operative visits. All of our doctors are top-notch and experienced with post-operative care and can answer any question you can think of.

If you really want to see only your surgeon, we are happy to arrange the appointment and give you directions.

My optometrist sent me for cataract surgery? Do I go back to that doctor?

For your final post-operative checkup, we usually send you back to your original optometric doctor. We are always happy to see you for ALL of your visits, but by this point, your eye has mostly healed and the final visit is mainly to double-check your ocular health and to measure you for potential glasses.

This is meant to be a convenience for you. Also, optometric doctors are excellent at refraction and will do a superb job tweaking your vision for glasses (if needed). We send your surgery information to your optometrist and we're always available to you if you have a problem or concern.

It's been several weeks since my surgery, and my vision STILL seems blurry. Is something wrong?

Corneal cloudiness improves at a different rate in everyone. It takes a while for some corneas to clear . . . this is especially true if you had a dense cataract, are over 70 years of age, or had pre-existing corneal disease like Fuchs' Dystrophy.

We all heal at different rates, and some people take a few weeks for things to sharpen.

Also, your blurry vision at this point might simply be a need for new glasses. We can perform the most "perfect cataract surgery in the world," but you may not see the full improvement until we put you in glasses (if you need them).

How soon can I get new glasses?

You will need to wait about three weeks after your cataract surgery to get glasses. This is because prescriptions tend to fluctuate immediately after surgery. If we prescribe glasses too soon, your prescription might not be stable, and would require you to get your glasses remade.

Can I wear my old glasses while I wait for my eye to heal?

Yes. You can wear your old pre-surgery glasses if they seem to help your vision. Even though the prescription is "wrong," it won't hurt your eyes to wear them. Some people actually pop a lens out of their frames as a temporary fix between surgeries. Our optical department can do that for you if you like.

I've never worn reading glasses before ... and now I need reading glasses?

If you used to be "nearsighted" before your surgery, you may never have needed readers or bifocals before ... you lucky dog! However, I bet your distance vision was pretty crummy!

Now that we've adjusted your eyes for better distance vision, you may be having a harder time seeing close up! For the first time in your life, you might actually require reading glasses!

Don't worry ... nothing has gone wrong with your surgery. Your eye "prescription" has simply changed. With cataract surgery, we have the opportunity to eliminate your nearsightedness and allow you to see better at distance. Most people love this improvement. Many of our patients tell us they can now see their television better without their spectacles. Many can drive a car without glasses. Others find it easier to navigate their homes as they can see across the room ... all without searching for glasses or putting in their contacts. Distance vision is a wonderful thing!

However, this improvement is not without some cost - to gain far focus, you must lose some near focus. Fortunately, reading glasses should fix everything, and most people enjoy the compromise.

I see clearer, but I am disappointed as I STILL need glasses for both distance and reading!

Unfortunately, with cataract surgery your eventual glasses prescription is not 100% predictable, and sometimes focus "surprises" like this happen. Fortunately, residual prescription is correctable with new spectacles or contacts. The goal of cataract surgery is to sharpen your vision, not necessarily to make you eyeglass-free. You will get used to your new prescription ... and in the end, hopefully, you'll appreciate that the improved visual "clarity" that you've gained outweighs your continued reliance on spectacles.

Colors seem different in my operated eye. Everything seems clearer and ... bluer!

This is a common observation. Most cataracts have a yellow-brown tint to them, and this can make colors seem dull and washed out. It's almost like there are blue-blocker sunglasses inside your eyeball!

When we removed the cataract, we replaced it with a clear implant. Afterward, you'll see more accurate colors, and objects can actually look bluer. This is how they are supposed to look! This color improvement will look even more impressive if you still have a cataract in your second eye to compare the difference with.

I am unimpressed with my visual improvements.

The decision to have cataract surgery is not always an easy or obvious one. Before surgery, we have a long discussion about the pros and cons of surgery ... and whether cataract surgery is "worth it." We tend to be conservative and don't like to perform surgery on someone unless we feel there will be a visual improvement.

Despite this counseling, every once in a while we'll encounter a case where the vision doesn't seem to be much better afterwards ... even after we've "maxed out" the vision with a new glasses prescription. Then the question becomes ... why?

Sometimes this is because of other pre-existing ocular problems like macular degeneration or diabetic damage that limits your best vision. Sometimes this is because dry eye or a poor tear-film creates optical aberrations that will slowly improve over many months. Sometimes, vision loss is from unknown aging changes in the eye that can't be detected or "fixed." Even with modern microscopy and high-tech imaging, subtle ocular disease can't always be detected ahead of time.

In fact, sometimes we don't truly know if you'll "see better" until AFTER your cataract is out. If you are underwhelmed with your vision after your first cataract surgery, we may want to delay your second eye and reassess whether the "visual benefits still outweigh the risks" of a second operation.

I read somewhere that Medicare will only pay for part of my glasses. What's that all about?

Normally, Medicare doesn't pay for glasses or contacts. However, after cataract surgery Medicare and some other insurances DO assist in the cost of frames and lenses. You should ask our optical department how this reimbursement works.

This is my second surgery and my vision seems blurrier than after the first! What's going on?

After surgery, everyone has blurriness. How MUCH blur seems to be different with everyone, even different between eyes. If your first eye cleared quickly, and your second eye is somewhat slower, then naturally you're going to be a little worried that something went wrong!

Try not to fret. This is the normal healing process, and your vision should clear up. We tend to perform surgery on your non-dominant eye first . . . and blurriness after your second surgery (on your dominant eye) tends to be more noticeable.

My second eye is doing great ... but my vision is not as impressive as after my first cataract operation!

Yes, this is likely true for two reasons:

1. We prefer to operate on the worse cataract first.

2. Going from two "bad eyes" to one "clear eye" after your first surgery tends to be more visually impressive than gaining two "clear eyes" after your second operation.

My second surgery went fine, but it seems like the operation took longer and there was a lot more going on!

We hear this comment a lot, and we think this observation has a lot to do with expectations.

Before your first surgery, you didn't know WHAT to expect, and you may have been pleasantly surprised at how easy and stress-free the procedure ended up being.

With the second eye, however, people tend to focus on what seems DIFFERENT. You might notice different steps during your procedure. If the eye seems more irritated, this seems a bigger deal! In addition, we used an analgesic during your first surgery that tends to make you forget! Don't worry, we perform cataract surgery the same each time!

I still have drops left over from my first surgery. Can I use them with my second surgery?

No, it's better to use a fresh set of drops if possible. All medications, even antibiotics, can be colonized by bacteria in the air or from your eyelashes during normal use. While rare, it's better to have a fresh set of drops and take no chances.

Can cataracts come back?

No, cataracts can't reform. The plastic implant that has replaced your cloudy lens is inert and will essentially last forever. That being said, sometimes a cloudiness called an "after cataract" can form.

This can happen months or years after successful cataract surgery. A film forms on the back of the plastic implant inside your eye. This film can obscure vision and can recreate many of your original cataract symptoms like blur or glare. This is not a complication and this cloudy film is common ... up to 30% of people will form this opacification, sometimes many years after a successful surgery.

If I develop one of these "after cataracts" am I going to need another surgery?

No, you will not need a surgery. This film can be fixed with a simpler procedure called a YAG Laser Capsulotomy. We use a laser to create a "hole" through the cloudy film.

This laser procedure is painless, takes only a few minutes, and you will not need eye drops afterwards because this is not truly a surgery. The visual improvement is often instantaneous. Once this "after cataract" has been dealt with, the film cannot come back.

Chapter 9

❧ Restrictions & Precautions ❧

Tomoka "Eye-Toons"

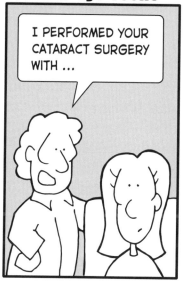

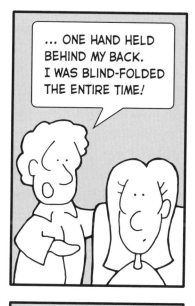

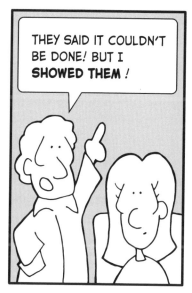

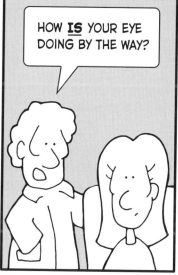

Restrictions & Precautions

Safety precautions after your operation

The key to a healthy recovery is common sense. Try to baby your eye during the first few weeks after your surgery. If you have any odd symptoms, call our office - we can work in emergency appointments very quickly and false alarms don't bother us! Better safe than sorry when it comes to eye surgery!

Can I drive?

You can drive whenever you feel you are seeing well enough to drive safely, but we recommend getting the "ok" from us first. You should bring a driver for your first post-operative checkup as your depth perception may be off. We'll check your vision after surgery to ensure you're seeing well enough to drive a car (most people are fine).

Many people have some light sensitivity after surgery. What we DON'T want you to do is start driving with a sensitive eye. Just use common sense, wear sunglasses, and take it easy at first.

How careful do I need to be with rubbing?

The day of your surgery, you need to be extremely gentle with your eye. Rubbing or poking the eye during the first few days can increase the chance for infection.

Now, don't get too worried at this point. If you accidentally forget and touch the eye, the sky won't fall down. As long as the vision is stable and you're not having pain, you'll be fine. Many people leave the clear shield over their eye that first day as a reminder, taking if off only to put in their eye drops.

It's okay to gently pat around the eyelids, as long as you are not pushing on the eyeball itself. One of your post-operative eye drops (the steroid) leaves behind a white residue that tends to collect in the corners of your eye. It is okay to gently wipe this buildup away with a tissue or Q-tip ... just don't push on the eyeball itself.

Do I have to wear the sunglasses all the time?

The sunglasses are entirely for your comfort. Many people have photophobia (sensitivity to light) after their surgery. Also, your pupil may be dilated for a few days and the sunglasses can make you more comfortable. Finally, it's nice to have something covering the eye immediately after surgery so that random objects (sand, bugs, rubber bands) don't hit you in the eye.

Is it OK to use the shower?

Yes, but keep water and soap out of your eye during the first week. Also, be careful in the shower if you are unsteady. Cataract surgery can throw off your depth perception... you do NOT want to slip or fall and hit your eye.

What are my physical restrictions? Can I exercise?

After surgery, the recovery time is pretty quick. Every surgeon has different opinions on exercise, so here is our preferred timeline of acceptable activity:

The day of surgery: Take it easy on the day of surgery. It's okay to walk around the house or even go out to dinner . . . as long as you pace yourself and don't build up a sweat from exertion.

After your one-day checkup: You can walk around and stay active during this first week. Take long walks, go to work, shop, chores - any light activity that doesn't tire you out or make you sweat profusely is fine. No weightlifting during this first week and try to avoid lifting heavy things (bags, purses, etc.) more than 20 pounds.

After your one-week checkup: Once we've gotten through the first week, we're mostly out of the danger zone for post-operative leaks or infection. You can increase your activity and start basic workouts.

After your three-week checkup: At this point, the healing process is nearly complete. It's okay to jog, lift, and perform aerobics.

The only activity restrictions at this point are no "ultra-exercise" for a few months. If you are a weightlifter, I would avoid heavy weights on full-body exercises (like squats, clean-and-jerk, and bent-over rows). Give your eyes a few more months to heal before running a marathon or competing in iron-man triathlons.

Can I golf?

After a week, it's usually safe to start golfing, as long as you use sensible precautions. Keep sweat and dirt out of your eyes, wear sunglasses, and do not let ANYTHING hit you in the eye. Take it easy with the heavy hitting and bend from the knee when picking up your ball or equipment.

Can I perform yard work?

We'd prefer you wait a week before messing around your yard or garden. Mowing can kick up dust and gardening involves a lot of bending over in dirt. We don't want you to get an infection from soil-based bacteria so try to curb your horticulture inclinations.

Is there any restriction with flying?

You shouldn't fly for a few days after surgery, but there isn't any real restrictions with flying as long as you're in a regular commercial airplane with pressurized cabins. No sky diving for one month.

When can I swim and use the hot tub?

We do not want you getting in a pool or hot tub for one week. Pool water contains many bacteria. No opening your eyes under water, no jumping off diving boards, and no canonballs to impress your friends, at least not for a little while.

Can I wear makeup?
It's okay to wear lipstick the day after surgery. However, do not use any eye makeup (eyeliner or mascara) for one week.

Can I get my hair done?
Yes, as long as reasonable precautions are made to keep dyes and chemicals away from your eye. This is especially important the week immediately after surgery.

I'm having flashes and floaters.
If you are having any odd symptoms, like new floaters in your vision, or flashing lights - call us. If your eye is hurting and your vision worsening - call us.

Something weird is happening to my eye?
If there is anything odd happening to your eye, call our office first. Even after office hours and the weekend, we have an on-call physician.

I'm very happy with my results!
Great! We're very happy for you! Cataract surgery is a wonderful operation that makes real improvements in people's lives and we feel blessed to be a part of this process.

Tomoka Eye is still growing, so feel free to refer your friends and add us to your will. You might also consider contributing to the Tomoka

Eye Foundation. This is a non-profit organization we created to help support our local children and seeing eye dog population.

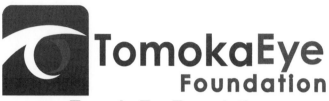

www.TomokaEyeFoundation.org

❧ Closing Remarks ❧

Tomoka "Eye-Toons"

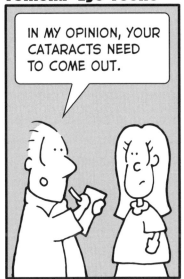

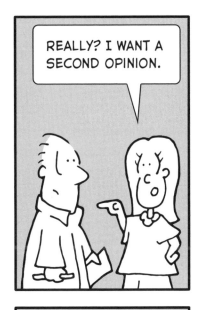

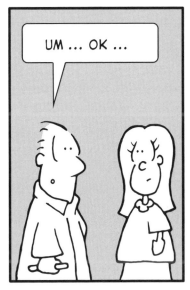

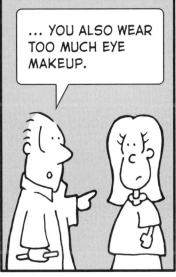

Thank you!

We hope you've found this book useful. There is a surprising amount of information within these pages and we hope you didn't find this overwhelming.

Cataract surgery is a wonderful surgery - it gives back clear vision, and modern techniques have made the procedure safer than ever.

If you still have questions about your cataract, contact our office and we'll make sure you get an answer. Good vision and happy results are the goal here and we want you to have a great outcome!

Thank you so much,
The Tomoka Eye Doctors

Tomoka "Eye-Toons"

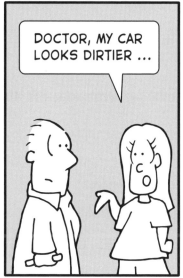

DOCTOR, MY CAR LOOKS DIRTIER ...

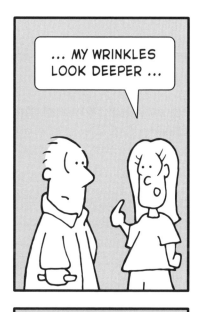

... MY WRINKLES LOOK DEEPER ...

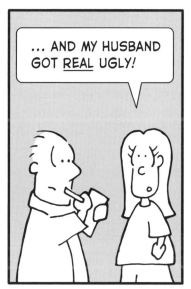

... AND MY HUSBAND GOT <u>REAL</u> UGLY!

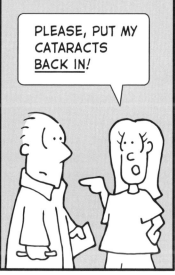

PLEASE, PUT MY CATARACTS <u>BACK IN</u>!

Directions to Surgery Center

The Tomoka Eye Surgery Center is located adjacent to our central Ormond Beach office. If you've never been there, here are directions and a map:

1. From I-95, get off at the SR-40 exit (EXIT 268)
This is the main Ormond exit. There is a Super Walmart near this exit.

2. Drive east (i.e., toward the beach) on Granada/ SR-40 for 1.6 miles
Granada Blvd. is the main road in Ormond Beach and is sometimes called State Road 40.

3. Turn right (south) onto Clyde Morris Blvd
There is a busy gas station at this intersection.

4. Drive south on Clyde Morris for one mile. Our office will be on your left.
Our office is on the left (east side of street) immediately after the Hand Avenue intersection. Our building looks like this from the street:

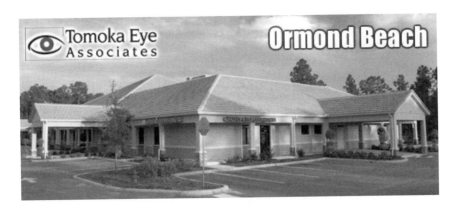

Tomoka Surgery Center
345 Clyde Morris Blvd., Suite 300
Ormond Beach, FL 32174

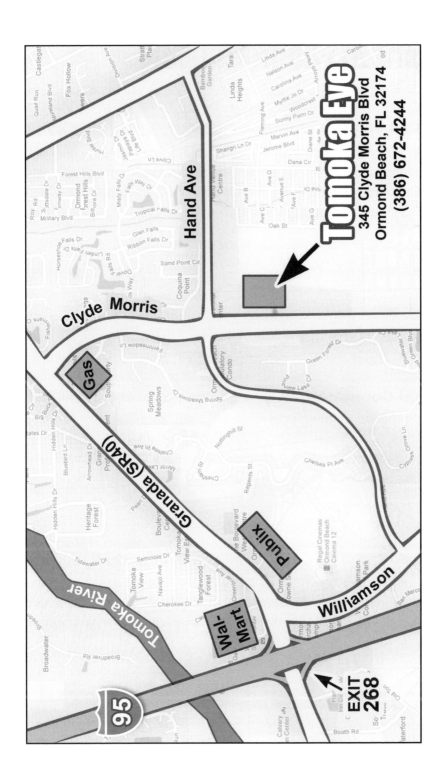

Important Phone Numbers

Tomoka Eye Main Number   (386) 672-4244

This is our central switchboard. Our calling center staff can track down anyone (including your doctor) on the weekend or nights if you are having an eye emergency. If you have any questions about ANYTHING, use this number and we'll route you to the correct person.

Tomoka Surgery Center   (386) 672-7575

If you need to call specifically about your surgery, this is our front desk staff. For example, this is who you'd call if you had a flat tire and were running late for surgery.

Surgical Coordinators   (386) 672-4244

Our main phone number can also be used to reach our surgery coordinators. They set up surgery, check calendars, look at your insurance, and can go over all the logistic details with you. If you have a question about your surgery or insurance coverage, this is the person to call.

Website   www.TomokaEye.com

Visit us online to learn more about Tomoka Eye and your doctors. You'll also find directions to each office, videos on common eye diseases, and office paperwork that you complete before your office visit.